APHRODISIAC HARVEST

Unveiling Nature's Potent Fruits
for Men's Libido

HAMZA FAGGE AHMAD

Cover design by: Mai Nama Designs

*This book is dedicated to all men in the world
fighting low libido/sex-drive and to all women
supporting their men to fight this battle.*

CONTENTS

INTRODUCTION

Welcome to a journey through the lush landscapes of Africa, where nature unfolds its secrets to enhance men's vitality and libido. In "Aphrodisiac Harvest," we explore the rich tapestry of natural fruits that have been revered for centuries for their potential to boost male libido. From the sun-kissed savannas to the dense rainforests, discover the bounty that Mother Nature provides to kindle the flames of passion.

CHAPTER 1: THE ESSENCE OF LIBIDO

Understanding Libido

In the heart of Africa, where vibrant cultures and diverse landscapes intertwine, the concept of libido holds profound significance. Libido, often referred to as sexual desire or passion, is a fundamental aspect of human nature. It goes beyond the physical, reaching into the realms of emotional connection and overall well-being.

The Holistic Nature Of Libido

Libido is not merely a physiological function but a complex interplay of physical, psychological, and social factors. In African traditions, the understanding of libido transcends the individual, emphasizing its connection to community, fertility, and the vitality of relationships. This holistic perspective forms the foundation for exploring the natural fruits that have, for generations, been believed to enhance this vital force.

Libido As A Reflection Of Health

A healthy libido is often considered an indicator of overall well-being. In African cultures, the ebb and flow of libido are seen as reflections of one's physical health, emotional balance, and spiritual vitality. This chapter sets the stage for our journey, inviting readers to appreciate libido not only as a personal aspect but as a harmonious expression of life's energies.

Cultural Perspectives

Aphrodisiac Traditions

Across the diverse cultures of Africa, the use of natural

aphrodisiacs has been woven into rituals, culinary traditions, and folk medicine. These traditions acknowledge the intimate connection between nature and human desire. From the deserts of North Africa to the rainforests of the Congo, the wisdom of using fruits to enhance libido has been passed down through generations.

Symbolism And Rituals

Fruits with aphrodisiac properties often carry symbolic meanings in various African cultures. Some are integrated into marriage ceremonies, symbolizing fertility and the promise of a passionate union. This chapter explores the rich tapestry of symbolism surrounding these fruits and how their inclusion in rituals reflects a cultural understanding of intimacy and connection.

Ancestral Wisdom

The knowledge of libido-enhancing fruits is deeply rooted in ancestral wisdom. Elders and healers in African communities have long recognized the benefits of specific fruits in promoting vitality and passion. This chapter delves into the role of ancestral wisdom in shaping cultural attitudes toward libido and the natural remedies that have stood the test of time.

As we embark on this journey through the orchards of Africa, we invite you to explore the essence of libido, deeply intertwined with cultural nuances and the natural abundance that the continent offers. The following chapters will unravel the secrets held within the succulent fruits that have, for centuries, been celebrated for their potential to ignite passion and enhance the vitality of men.

CHAPTER 2: BAOBAB BLISS

The Baobab Miracle

The Grandeur of Baobab

Our journey into the realm of natural aphrodisiacs leads us to the majestic baobab tree, an icon of African landscapes. With its massive trunk and unique silhouette, the baobab is more than a tree; it's a symbol of life, resilience, and natural wonder. This chapter explores the baobab's remarkable qualities and its historical significance in the cultural tapestry of Africa.

Nutritional Powerhouse

Unlock the nutritional treasure trove concealed within the baobab fruit. Packed with essential vitamins and minerals, baobab is a potent natural supplement that contributes to overall health. Dive into the rich content of vitamin C, antioxidants, and other nutrients that not only boost the immune system but also play a crucial role in supporting reproductive health and libido.

Vitamin C Boost

Libido and Immune Health

Discover the intimate connection between vitamin C and libido. As a powerful antioxidant, vitamin C not only strengthens the immune system but also supports the production of hormones essential for sexual health. Unravel the dual benefits of baobab as a fruit that not only invigorates but also nourishes, providing a holistic approach to well-being.

Baobab Rituals

Delve into cultural practices that incorporate baobab into rituals celebrating fertility and vitality. From traditional ceremonies to everyday culinary traditions, baobab has been a staple in African communities, symbolizing the abundance of life. Learn how the wisdom of using baobab has been passed down through generations, connecting communities to the essence of nature.

As we stand beneath the sprawling branches of the baobab tree, we witness the convergence of cultural reverence and nutritional richness. Join us in the next chapter as we explore another fruit that holds the promise of passion and vitality in the diverse landscapes of Africa.

CHAPTER 3:
HEAVENLY DATES

Nature's Candy

The Allure of Dates

Our exploration of natural aphrodisiacs leads us to the enchanting world of dates—a fruit revered for its sweetness and sensory indulgence. Dates often referred to as nature's candy, have played a central role in culinary traditions and rituals across Africa. In this chapter, we unravel the irresistible charm of dates and their historical significance in kindling the flames of passion.

Date Palms: Oasis of Sensuality

Step into the oasis of date palms, where the air is infused with the sweet aroma of ripening fruit. Date palms, with their towering presence and clusters of succulent dates, symbolize abundance and fertility. Learn about the cultural symbolism of date palms and how they have been integrated into ceremonies celebrating love, marriage, and sensuality.

Energy Elixirs

Nutrient-Rich Delights

Dates, beyond their delectable taste, are a powerhouse of nutrients. Rich in natural sugars, fiber, and essential vitamins and minerals, dates provide a quick and sustained energy boost.

Explore the nutritional composition of dates and how these energy elixirs contribute to vitality, stamina, and overall well-being.

Historical Aphrodisiac

Uncover the historical use of dates as natural aphrodisiacs in various cultures. From ancient Egypt to the Arabian Peninsula, dates have been revered for their potential to enhance libido and foster intimacy. Delve into historical anecdotes and cultural practices that highlight the significance of dates in the realm of passion.

Culinary Sensuality

Date-Inspired Delicacies

Embark on a culinary journey as we explore the diverse ways dates are incorporated into tantalizing dishes. From sweet treats to savory delights, discover how dates add a touch of sensuality to traditional recipes. Learn about date-inspired delicacies that have been crafted to celebrate love and intimacy.

Rituals of Connection

Dates, in their natural sweetness, have become a symbol of connection and shared moments. This chapter explores rituals and customs that involve the sharing of dates, fostering a sense of closeness and bonding. From romantic encounters to communal celebrations, dates become more than a fruit—they become a catalyst for shared joy and connection.

CHAPTER 4: MARVELOUS MANGOES

Tropical Sensuality

Mangoes: Nature's Aphrodisiac

Our exploration of natural aphrodisiacs brings us to the sun-kissed realms of mango orchards. Mangoes, with their luscious sweetness and tropical allure, have captured the hearts and palates of people across Africa. In this chapter, we delve into the marvelous world of mangoes—a fruit celebrated not only for its taste but also for its potential to kindle the flames of passion.

Mango Orchards: Havens of Romance

Step into the vibrant landscapes where mango orchards thrive. These lush havens are not just sources of delicious fruit but are also imbued with a sense of romance. Discover how mango orchards become settings for romantic encounters, celebrations of love, and rituals symbolizing fertility and sensuality.

Vitamins and Minerals

Nutritional Elegance

Beyond their sumptuous flavor, mangoes boast a nutritional profile that contributes to overall well-being. Rich in vitamins A, C, and E, as well as minerals like zinc, mangoes play a vital role in supporting immune health and reproductive function. Uncover the nutritional elegance that makes mangoes a natural elixir for vitality.

The Sensual Impact of Vitamins

Explore how the vitamins in mangoes, particularly vitamin E, contribute to skin health and may have a sensual impact. Vitamin E is known for its antioxidant properties, promoting circulation and supporting the health of reproductive organs. Delve into the science behind these sensual benefits and the cultural significance attached to mangoes.

CHAPTER 5: AVOCADO ARDOR

Creamy Euphoria

The Allure of Avocados

Our exploration of natural aphrodisiacs leads us to the velvety embrace of avocados. Avocados, with their creamy texture and rich taste, have transcended their status as a culinary delight to become symbols of sensuality. In this chapter, we delve into the allure of avocados—a fruit that not only tantalizes the taste buds but also holds the promise of enhancing male vitality and passion.

Nutrient-Rich Powerhouse

Unlock the nutritional wealth concealed within the green goodness of avocados. Packed with heart-healthy monounsaturated fats, vitamins E, B6, and folate, as well as minerals like potassium, avocados contribute to overall well-being. Explore the nutritional powerhouse that positions avocados as a natural elixir for vitality.

Healthy Fats for Hormones

The Role of Healthy Fats

Delve into the significance of healthy fats in avocados, particularly monounsaturated fats, and their impact on hormone production. Discover how these fats contribute to the synthesis of hormones essential for reproductive health. Gain insights into the interconnected relationship between nutrition, hormones, and overall well-being.

Culinary Symphony

Explore the diverse ways avocados harmonize with culinary creations. From silky smooth guacamole to avocado-infused desserts, the culinary world celebrates the versatility of avocados. Learn about mouthwatering recipes that not only showcase the culinary appeal of avocados but also invite sensuality to the dining experience.

CHAPTER 6: SUCCULENT WATERMELON

Juicy Indulgence

The Temptation of Watermelons

Our journey into the world of natural aphrodisiacs brings us to the succulent realms of watermelon orchards. Watermelons, with their refreshing juiciness and vibrant hue, stand as symbols of summer delight. In this chapter, we explore the juicy indulgence of watermelons—a fruit that not only quenches thirst but also holds the promise of enhancing male vitality and passion.

Citrulline Magic

Dive into the science behind watermelon's aphrodisiac properties, particularly the presence of citrulline. Citrulline, an amino acid, is known for its potential to boost blood flow, contributing to improved circulation. Uncover the citrulline magic within watermelons and how this natural compound may have positive implications for male reproductive health.

CHAPTER 7: PASSIONATE PAPAYAS

Tropical Passion

Our exploration of natural aphrodisiacs takes us to the tropical charm of papayas. Papayas, with their vibrant color and luscious taste, have long been associated with exotic indulgence. In this chapter, we delve into the tropical passion of papayas—a fruit that not only delights the palate but also holds the promise of enhancing male vitality and passion.

Enzymes for Endurance

Explore the enzymatic wonders within papayas, particularly papain and chymopapain. These enzymes are believed to aid digestion and have potential benefits for overall well-being. Uncover how the unique combination of nutrients and enzymes in papayas contributes to endurance, both in the culinary realm and, some believe, in matters of passion.

Cultural Significance

Delve into the cultural significance of papayas in various tropical regions. From symbolic representations in art to the inclusion of papayas in traditional rituals, this chapter explores how papayas have become intertwined with cultural expressions of love, sensuality, and fertility.

CHAPTER 8: ZESTY CITRUS FRUITS

Citrus Symphony

The Zesty Allure of Citrus

Our exploration of natural aphrodisiacs takes a zesty turn as we delve into the world of citrus fruits. Oranges, lemons, grapefruits, and limes bring a burst of freshness and tanginess that invigorates the senses. In this chapter, we explore the citrus symphony—a medley of flavors that not only tantalizes the taste buds but also holds the promise of enhancing male vitality and passion.

Vitamin C Surge

Dive into the abundance of vitamin C found in citrus fruits and its impact on immune health and overall well-being. Beyond its well-known role in supporting the immune system, vitamin C contributes to the health of blood vessels and may have implications for male reproductive health. Uncover the vitamin C surge within citrus fruits and how it adds a refreshing dimension to their aphrodisiac allure.

CHAPTER 9: MYSTERIOUS MORINGA

Green Vitality

Our exploration of natural aphrodisiacs takes us to the green landscapes where moringa thrives. Moringa, with its nutrient-rich leaves and versatile applications, stands as a symbol of green vitality. In this chapter, we delve into the mysterious world of moringa—a plant that not only nourishes the body but also holds the promise of enhancing male vitality and passion.

Nutrient-Rich Powerhouse

Unlock the nutritional wealth concealed within moringa leaves. Packed with vitamins, minerals, and antioxidants, moringa is a nutritional powerhouse that supports overall health. Explore the unique combination of nutrients in moringa and how it contributes to vitality, energy, and potentially, aspects of reproductive health.

Cultural Significance

Delve into the cultural significance of moringa in regions where it has been traditionally consumed. From medicinal uses to symbolic representations, moringa holds a special place in the cultural tapestry of certain communities. This chapter explores the cultural nuances associated with moringa and its role in traditional practices.

CHAPTER 10: POWERFUL PINEAPPLES

Tropical Elixir

The Tangy Sweetness of Pineapples

Our journey through the world of natural aphrodisiacs culminates in the tropical embrace of pineapples. Pineapples, with their tangy sweetness and distinctive crown, stand as symbols of exotic indulgence. In this final chapter, we explore the tropical elixir of pineapples—a fruit that not only delights the palate but also holds the promise of enhancing male vitality and passion.

Bromelain Benefits

Dive into the unique enzyme found in pineapples—bromelain—and its potential benefits for digestive health. Beyond its digestive properties, bromelain is believed by some to have positive effects on circulation and inflammation. Uncover the bromelain benefits within pineapples and how this enzyme adds a tantalizing layer to their aphrodisiac allure.

Cultural Symbolism

Delve into the cultural symbolism of pineapples in various tropical regions. From expressions of hospitality to representations in art and folklore, pineapples carry cultural significance that transcends their culinary appeal. This chapter explores how pineapples have become intertwined with cultural expressions of love, warmth, and celebration.

CONCLUSION: A TAPESTRY OF APHRODISIACS

As we conclude our exploration of natural fruits that increase men's libido in Africa, we have journeyed through lush landscapes, tasted exotic flavors, and uncovered the cultural tapestry that weaves these fruits into the fabric of life. The tangy sweetness of pineapples serves as a fitting conclusion to a rich and diverse array of aphrodisiacs.

This journey invites you to embrace not only the culinary delights but also the cultural and historical narratives that surround these fruits. From the baobab's resilience to the dates' historical allure, from the mango's tropical charm to the avocado's creamy indulgence, each fruit adds a unique note to the symphony of aphrodisiacs.

May this exploration inspire a deeper appreciation for the connection between nature, culture, and the pursuit of passion. As you savor the tangy sweetness of pineapples, let it be a reminder that the richness of life's experiences is enhanced by the diverse and vibrant tapestry of the natural world.

Cheers to the tantalizing world of aphrodisiacs, and may your journey through passion and vitality continue to unfold in harmony with the gifts that nature generously provides.

RECIPES FOR YOU!

1. Avocado And Berry Smoothie:

Ingredients:

1 ripe avocado

1 cup mixed berries (strawberries, blueberries, raspberries)

1 banana

1 cup spinach (fresh or frozen)

1 cup almond milk

Instructions:

Blend all ingredients until smooth. Avocado provides healthy fats, while berries offer antioxidants.

2. Mango and Maca Smoothie:

Ingredients:

1 cup mango chunks (fresh or frozen)

1 tablespoon maca powder

1/2 cup Greek yogurt

1 tablespoon honey

1 cup coconut water

Instructions:

Blend all ingredients. Mango brings natural sweetness, and maca is believed to support energy and stamina.

3. Pineapple and Ginger Infused Water:

Ingredients:

1 cup pineapple chunks

1 tablespoon grated ginger

1 liter water

Instructions:

Combine pineapple and ginger in water. Allow to infuse for a few hours. Pineapple contains bromelain, while ginger supports circulation.

4. Salmon with Avocado Salsa:

Ingredients:

Grilled salmon fillets

1 ripe avocado, diced

1/2 red onion, finely chopped

Fresh cilantro, chopped

Lime juice

Instructions:

Mix avocado, onion, cilantro, and lime juice for a salsa. Serve over grilled salmon. Salmon provides omega-3 fatty acids.

5. Date and Walnut Energy Bites:

Ingredients:

1 cup dates, pitted

1 cup walnuts

1 tablespoon chia seeds

1 teaspoon cinnamon

Instructions:

Blend dates and walnuts until a dough forms. Add chia seeds and cinnamon. Roll into small energy bites. Dates are known for their energy-boosting properties.

6. Watermelon and Feta Salad:

Ingredients:

Cubed watermelon

Feta cheese

Mint leaves, chopped

Balsamic glaze

Instructions:

Mix watermelon, feta, and mint. Drizzle with balsamic glaze. Watermelon contains citrulline, linked to improved blood flow.

7. Moringa Green Smoothie:

Ingredients:

1 cup pineapple chunks

Handful of spinach

1 tablespoon moringa powder

1/2 banana

Coconut water

Instructions:

Blend pineapple, spinach, moringa powder, banana, and coconut water. Moringa is rich in nutrients.

8. Lemon Garlic Shrimp Pasta:

Ingredients:

Whole-grain pasta

Shrimp, peeled and deveined

Garlic, minced

Lemon juice

Olive oil

Instructions:

Cook pasta. Sauté shrimp and garlic in olive oil. Toss with cooked pasta. Lemon and garlic are associated with vitality.

9. Chicken and Broccoli Stir-Fry:

Ingredients:

Chicken breast, thinly sliced

Broccoli florets

Soy sauce

Ginger, minced

Brown rice

Instructions:

Stir-fry chicken and broccoli in soy sauce and ginger. Serve over brown rice. Ginger is believed to support circulation.

10. Chocolate-Covered Strawberries:

Ingredients:

Fresh strawberries

Dark chocolate, melted

Instructions:

Dip strawberries in melted dark chocolate. Dark chocolate contains flavonoids associated with increased blood flow.

Remember to consult with a healthcare professional or nutritionist before making significant changes to your diet, especially if you have existing health conditions. These recipes aim to incorporate ingredients that are commonly believed to support vitality and libido, but individual responses may vary.

ABOUT THE AUTHOR

Hamza Ahmad Fagge is an aspiring writer and traditional healthcare & marriage consultant from Kano State, Nigeria with a vast experience in the field of fruits usage for health of more than 6 years.